Mediterranean Ketogenic Diet

The Essential Mediterranean
Cookbook for Weight Loss,
Regain Confidence and
Heal Your Body

Tilly Heather

Copyright © 2021 Tilly Heather

Table of content

1. Asparagus Salad with Oranges, Feta, and Hazelnuts
(serves 6)

Ingredients:

PESTO
1 teaspoon grated lemon zest plus 2 teaspoons juice
1 garlic clove, minced
Salt and pepper
½ cup extra-virgin olive oil
2 cups fresh mint leaves
¼ cup fresh basil leaves
¼ cup grated Pecorino Romano cheese

SALAD
4 ounces feta cheese, crumbled (1 cup)
¾ cup hazelnuts, toasted, skinned, and chopped
2 pounds asparagus, trimmed
2 oranges
Salt and pepper

Directions:

1. FOR THE PESTO Process mint, basil, Pecorino, lemon zest and juice, garlic, and ¾ teaspoon salt in food processor until finely chopped, about 20 seconds, scraping down sides of bowl as needed. Transfer to large bowl. Stir in oil and season with salt and pepper to taste.

2. FOR THE SALAD Cut asparagus tips from stalks into ¾-inch-long pieces. Slice asparagus stalks ⅛ inch thick on bias into approximate 2-inch lengths. Cut away peel and pith from oranges. Holding fruit over bowl, use paring knife to

slice between membranes to release segments. Add asparagus tips and stalks, orange segments, feta, and hazelnuts to pesto and toss to combine. Season with salt and pepper to taste. Serve.

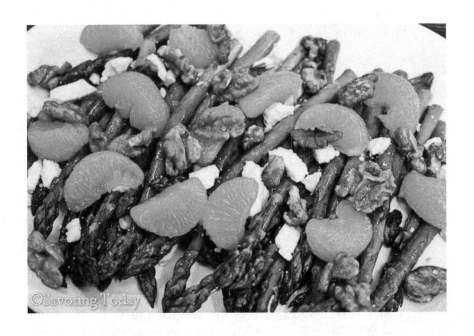

2. Roasted Beet and Carrot Salad with Cumin and Pistachios
(serves 6)

Ingredients:

1 small shallot, minced
1 teaspoon honey
½ teaspoon ground cumin
½ cup shelled pistachios, toasted and chopped
2 tablespoons minced fresh parsley
1 pound beets, trimmed
1 pound carrots, peeled and sliced on bias ¼ inch thick
2½ tablespoons extra-virgin olive oil
Salt and pepper
1 tablespoon grated lemon zest plus 3 tablespoons juice

Directions:

1. Adjust oven racks to middle and lowest positions. Place rimmed baking sheet on lower rack and heat oven to 450 degrees.

2. Wrap beets individually in aluminum foil and place in second rimmed baking sheet. Toss carrots with 1 tablespoon oil, ½ teaspoon salt, and ½ teaspoon pepper.

3. Working quickly, arrange carrots in single layer in hot baking sheet and place baking sheet with beets on middle rack. Roast until carrots are tender and well browned on 1 side, 20 to 25 minutes, and skewer inserted into center of beets meets little resistance (you will need to unwrap beets to test them), 35 to 45 minutes.

4. Carefully open foil packets and let beets sit until cool enough to handle. Carefully rub off beet skins using paper

towel. Slice beets into ½-inch-thick wedges, and, if large, cut in half crosswise.

5. Whisk lemon juice, shallot, honey, cumin, ¼ teaspoon salt, and ⅛ teaspoon pepper together in large bowl. Whisking constantly, slowly drizzle in remaining 1½ tablespoons oil. Add beets and carrots, toss to coat, and let cool to room temperature, about 20 minutes.

6. Add pistachios, parsley, and lemon zest to bowl with beets and carrots and toss to coat

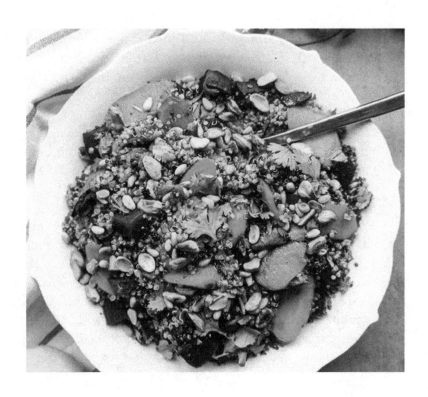

3. Green Bean Salad with Cilantro Sauce
(serves 8)

Ingredients:

2½ cups fresh cilantro leaves and stems, tough stem ends
trimmed (about 2 bunches)
½ cup extra-virgin olive oil
4 teaspoons lemon juice
1 scallion, sliced thin
¼ cup walnuts
2 garlic cloves, unpeeled
Salt and pepper
2 pounds green beans, trimmed

Directions:

1. Cook walnuts and garlic in 8-inch skillet over medium heat,
    stirring often, until toasted and fragrant, 5 to 7 minutes;
    transfer to bowl. Let garlic cool slightly, then peel and
    roughly chop.

2. Process walnuts, garlic, cilantro, oil, lemon juice, scallion, ½
    teaspoon salt, and ⅛ teaspoon pepper in food processor
    until smooth, about 1 minute, scraping down sides of bowl
    as needed; transfer to large bowl.

3. Bring 4 quarts water to boil in large pot over high heat.
    Meanwhile, fill large bowl halfway with ice and water. Add 1
    tablespoon salt and green beans to boiling water and cook
    until crisp-tender, 3 to 5 minutes. Drain green beans,
    transfer to ice water, and let sit until chilled, about 2
    minutes. Transfer green beans to bowl with cilantro sauce
    and gently toss until coated. Season with salt and pepper to
    taste. Serve. (Salad can be refrigerated for up to 3 hours.)

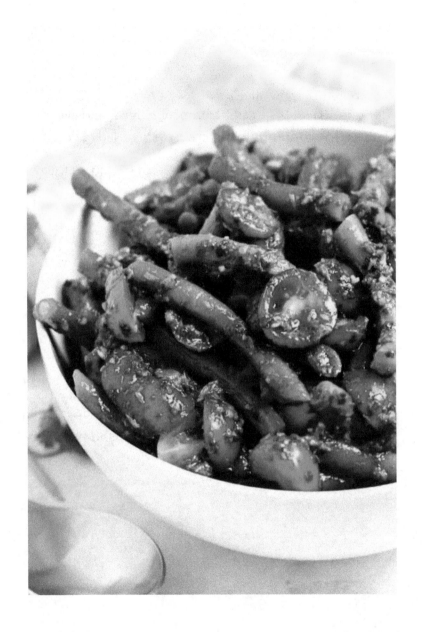

4. Brussels Sprout Salad with Pecorino and Pine Nuts
(serves 4)

Ingredients:

¼ cup extra-virgin olive oil
1 pound Brussels sprouts, trimmed, halved, and sliced very thin
2 ounces Pecorino Romano cheese, shredded (⅔ cup)
¼ cup pine nuts, toasted
Passi di: America's Test Kitchen. "The Complete Mediterranean Cookbook". iBooks.
1 small shallot, minced
1 garlic clove, minced
Salt and pepper
2 tablespoons lemon juice
1 tablespoon Dijon mustard

Directions:

Whisk lemon juice, mustard, shallot, garlic, and ½ teaspoon salt together in large bowl. Whisking constantly, slowly drizzle in oil. Add Brussels sprouts, toss to coat, and let sit for at least 30 minutes or up to 2 hours. Stir in Pecorino and pine nuts. Season with salt and pepper to taste. Serve.

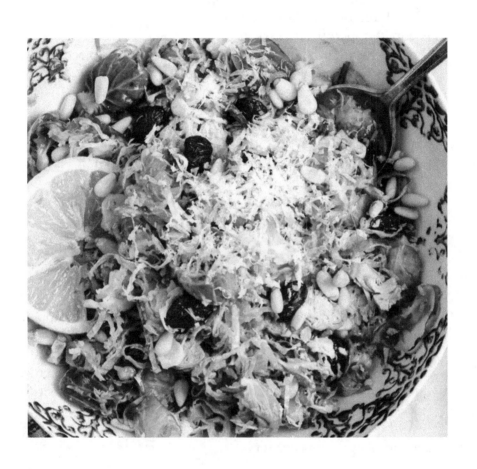

5. Mediterranean Chopped Salad
(serves 4)

Ingredients:

½ cup pitted kalamata olives, chopped
½ small red onion, chopped fine
½ cup chopped fresh parsley
1 romaine lettuce heart (6 ounces), cut into ½-inch pieces
4 ounces feta cheese, crumbled (1 cup)
3 tablespoons red wine vinegar
1 garlic clove, minced
3 tablespoons extra-virgin olive oil
1 (15-ounce) can chickpeas, rinsed
1 cucumber, peeled, halved lengthwise, seeded, and cut into ½-inch pieces
10 ounces grape tomatoes, quartered
Salt and pepper

Directions:

1. Toss cucumber and tomatoes with 1 teaspoon salt and let drain in colander for 15 minutes.
2. Whisk vinegar and garlic together in large bowl. Whisking constantly, slowly drizzle in oil. Add cucumber-tomato mixture, chickpeas, olives, onion, and parsley and toss to coat. Let sit for at least 5 minutes or up to 20 minutes.
3. Add lettuce and feta and gently toss to combine. Season with salt and pepper to taste. Serve.

6. Creamy Turkish Nut Dip
(makes 2 cups)

Ingredients:

"1 slice hearty white sandwich bread, crusts removed, torn into 1-inch pieces
¾ cup water, plus extra as needed
1 cup blanched almonds, blanched hazelnuts, pine nuts, or walnuts, toasted
¼ cup extra-virgin olive oil
2 tablespoons lemon juice, plus extra as needed
1 small garlic clove, minced
Salt and pepper
Pinch cayenne pepper"

Directions:

1. With fork, mash bread and water together in bowl into paste. Process bread mixture, nuts, oil, lemon juice, garlic, ½ teaspoon salt, ⅛ teaspoon pepper, and cayenne in blender until smooth, about 2 minutes. Add extra water as needed until sauce is barely thicker than consistency of heavy cream.

2. Season with salt, pepper, and extra lemon juice to taste. Serve at room temperature. (Sauce can be refrigerated for up to 2 days; bring to room temperature before serving.)

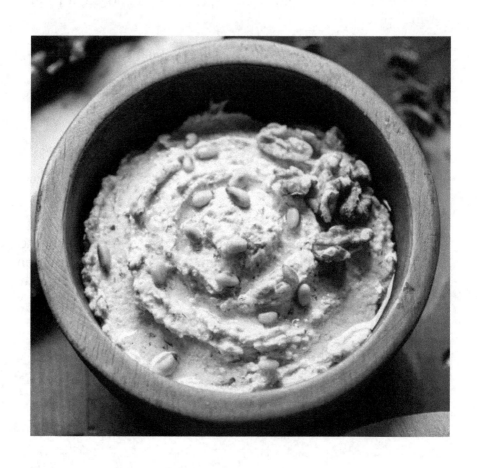

7. Provençal Anchovy Dip
(makes 1½ cups)

Ingredients:

¾ cup whole blanched almonds
20 anchovy fillets (1½ ounces), rinsed, patted dry, and minced
¼ cup water
2 tablespoons raisins
2 tablespoons lemon juice, plus extra for serving
1 garlic clove, minced
1 teaspoon Dijon mustard
Salt and pepper
¼ cup extra-virgin olive oil, plus extra for serving
1 tablespoon minced fresh

Directions:

1. Bring 4 cups water to boil in medium saucepan over medium-high heat. Add almonds and cook until softened, about 20 minutes. Drain and rinse well.

2. Process drained almonds, anchovies, water, raisins, lemon juice, garlic, mustard, ¼ teaspoon pepper, and ⅛ teaspoon salt in food processor to mostly smooth paste, about 2 minutes, scraping down sides of bowl as needed. With processor running, slowly add oil and process to smooth puree, about 2 minutes.

3. Transfer mixture to bowl, stir in 2 teaspoons chives, and season with salt and extra lemon juice to taste. (Dip can be refrigerated for up to 2 days; bring to room temperature before serving.) Sprinkle with remaining 1 teaspoon chives and drizzle with extra oil to taste before serving.

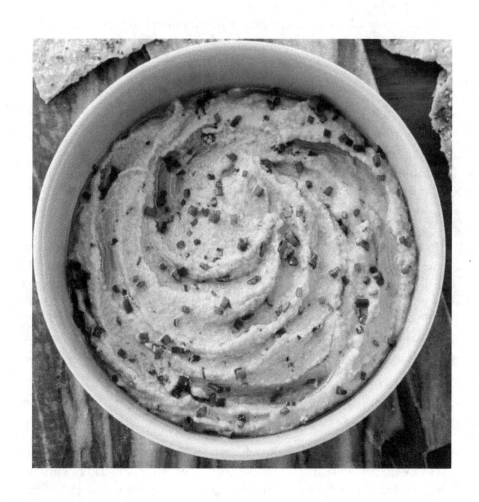

8. Lavash Crackers
(serves 12)

Ingredients:

1½ cups (8⅝ ounces) semolina flour
¾ cup (4⅛ ounces) whole-wheat flour
¾ cup (3¾ ounces) all-purpose flour
¾ teaspoon salt
1 cup warm water
⅓ cup extra-virgin olive oil, plus extra for brushing
1 large egg, lightly beaten
2 tablespoons sesame seeds
2 teaspoons sea salt or kosher salt
1 teaspoon coarsely ground pepper

Directions:

1. Using stand mixer fitted with dough hook, mix semolina flour, whole-wheat flour, all-purpose flour, and salt together on low speed. Gradually add water and oil and knead until dough is smooth and elastic, 7 to 9 minutes. Turn dough out onto lightly floured counter and knead by hand to form smooth, round ball. Divide dough into 4 equal pieces, brush with oil, and cover with plastic wrap. Let rest at room temperature for 1 hour.

2. Adjust oven racks to upper-middle and lower-middle positions and heat oven to 425 degrees. Lightly coat two 18 by 13-inch rimless (or inverted) baking sheets with vegetable oil spray.

3. Working with 2 pieces of dough (keep remaining dough covered with plastic), press dough into small rectangles, then transfer to prepared sheets. Using rolling pin and hands, roll and stretch dough evenly to edges of sheet. Using fork, poke holes in doughs at 2-inch intervals. Brush doughs with beaten egg,

then sprinkle each with 1½ teaspoons sesame seeds, ½ teaspoon salt, and ¼ teaspoon pepper. Press gently on seasonings to help them adhere.

4. Bake crackers until deeply golden brown, 15 to 18 minutes, switching and rotating sheets halfway through baking. Transfer crackers to wire rack and let cool completely. Let baking sheets cool completely before rolling out and baking remaining dough. Break cooled lavash into large crackers and serve. (Lavash can be stored at room temperature for up to 2 weeks.)

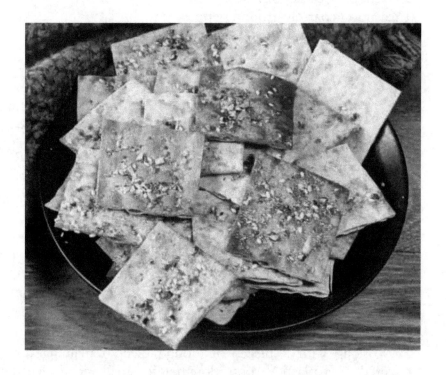

9. Marinated Green and Black Olives
(serves 8)

Ingredients:

1 cup brine-cured green olives with pits
1 cup brine-cured black olives with pits
¾ cup extra-virgin olive oil
1 shallot, minced
1 garlic clove, minced
2 teaspoons grated lemon zest
2 teaspoons minced fresh thyme
2 teaspoons minced fresh oregano
½ teaspoon red pepper flakes
½ teaspoon salt

Directions:

Rinse olives thoroughly, then drain and pat dry with paper towels. Toss olives with remaining ingredients in bowl, cover, and refrigerate for at least 4 hours or up to 4 days. Let sit at room temperature for at least 30 minutes before serving

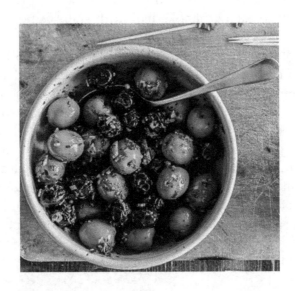

10. Marinated Artichokes
(serves 6)

Ingredients:

2 lemons
2½ cups extra-virgin olive oil
3 pounds baby artichokes (2 to 4 ounces each)
8 garlic cloves, peeled, 6 cloves smashed, 2 cloves minced
¼ teaspoon red pepper flakes
2 sprigs fresh thyme
Salt and pepper
2 tablespoons minced fresh mint

Directions:

1. Using vegetable peeler, remove three 2-inch strips zest from 1 lemon. Grate ½ teaspoon zest from second lemon and set aside. Halve and juice lemons to yield ¼ cup juice, reserving spent lemon halves.
2. Combine oil and lemon zest strips in large saucepan. Working with 1 artichoke at a time, cut top quarter off each artichoke, snap off outer leaves, and trim away dark parts. Peel and trim stem, then cut artichoke in half lengthwise (quarter artichoke if large). Rub each artichoke half with spent lemon half and place in saucepan.
3. Add smashed garlic, pepper flakes, thyme sprigs, 1 teaspoon salt, and ¼ teaspoon pepper to saucepan and bring to rapid simmer over high heat. Reduce heat to medium-low and simmer, stirring occasionally to submerge all artichokes, until artichokes can be pierced with fork but are still firm, "about 5 minutes. Remove from heat, cover, and let sit until artichokes are fork-tender and fully cooked, about 20 minutes.
4. Gently stir in ½ teaspoon reserved grated lemon zest, ¼ cup reserved lemon juice, and minced garlic. Transfer artichokes and oil to serving bowl and let cool to room temperature. Season with salt to taste and sprinkle with mint. Serve. (Artichokes and oil can be refrigerated for up to 4 days.)

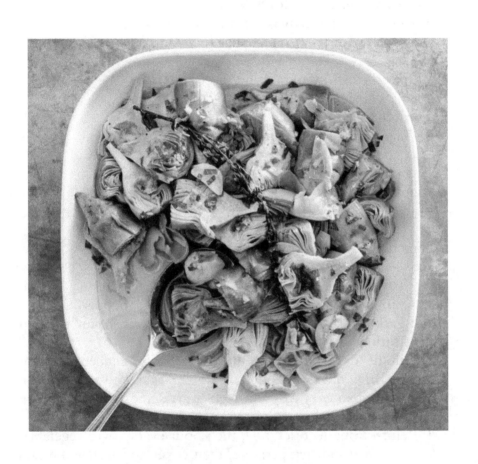

11. Giardiniera
(makes 1 pint)

Ingredients:

½ head cauliflower (1 pound), cored and cut into ½-inch florets
3 carrots, peeled and sliced ¼ inch thick on bias
3 celery ribs, cut crosswise into ½-inch pieces
1 red bell pepper, stemmed, seeded, and cut into ½-inch-wide strips
2 serrano chiles, stemmed and sliced thin
4 garlic cloves, sliced thin
1 cup chopped fresh dill
2¾ cups white wine vinegar
2¼ cups water
¼ cup sugar
2 tablespoons salt

Directions:

1. Combine cauliflower, carrots, celery, bell pepper, serranos, and garlic in large bowl, then transfer to four 1-pint jars with tight-fitting lids.
2. Bundle dill in cheesecloth and tie with kitchen twine to secure. Bring dill sachet, vinegar, water, sugar, and salt to boil in large saucepan over medium-high heat. Remove from heat and let steep for 10 minutes. Discard dill sachet.
3. Return brine to brief boil, then pour evenly over vegetables. Let cool to room temperature, then cover and refrigerate until vegetables taste pickled, at least 7 days or up to 1 month.

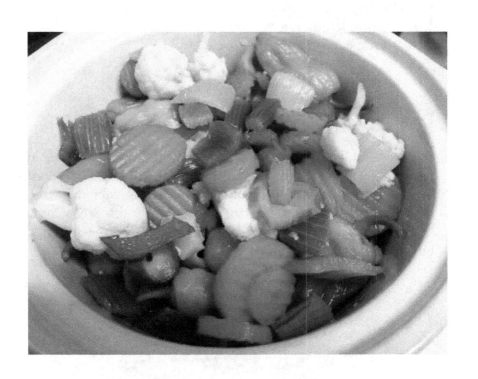

12. Spicy Whipped Feta with Roasted Red Peppers
(makes 2 cups)

Ingredients:

8 ounces feta cheese, crumbled (2 cups)
1 cup jarred roasted red peppers, rinsed, patted dry, and chopped
⅓ cup extra-virgin olive oil, plus extra for serving
1 tablespoon lemon juice
½ teaspoon cayenne pepper
¼ teaspoon pepper"

Directions:

1 Process feta, red peppers, oil, lemon juice, cayenne, and pepper in food processor until smooth, about 30 seconds, scraping down sides of bowl as needed. Transfer mixture to serving bowl, drizzle with extra oil to taste, and serve. (Dip can be refrigerated for up to 2 days; bring to room temperature before serving.)

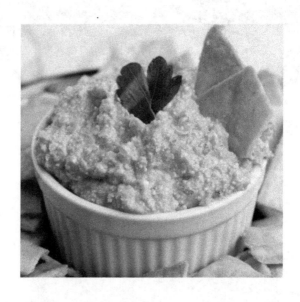

13. Broiled Feta with Olive Oil and Parsley
(serves 12)

Ingredients:

2 (8-ounce) blocks feta cheese, sliced into ½-inch-thick slabs
¼ teaspoon red pepper flakes
¼ teaspoon pepper
2 tablespoons extra-virgin olive oil
2 teaspoons minced fresh parsley

Directions:

Adjust oven rack 4 inches from broiler element and heat broiler. Pat feta dry with paper towels and arrange in broiler-safe gratin dish. Sprinkle with red pepper flakes and pepper. Broil until edges of cheese are golden, 3 to 8 minutes. Drizzle with oil, sprinkle with parsley, and serve immediately.

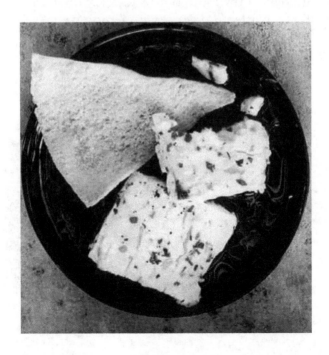

14. Pan-Fried Halloumi
(serves 6)

Ingredients:

2 tablespoons extra-virgin olive oil
Lemon wedges
2 tablespoons cornmeal
1 tablespoon all-purpose flour
1 (8-ounce) block halloumi cheese, sliced into ½-inch-thick slabs10. Marinated Green and Black Olives

Directions:

1. Combine cornmeal and flour in shallow dish. Working with 1 piece of cheese at a time, coat both wide sides with cornmeal mixture, pressing to help coating adhere; transfer to plate.
2. Heat oil in 12-inch nonstick skillet over medium heat until shimmering. Arrange halloumi in single layer in skillet and cook until golden brown on both sides, 2 to 4 minutes per side. Transfer to platter and serve with lemon wedges.

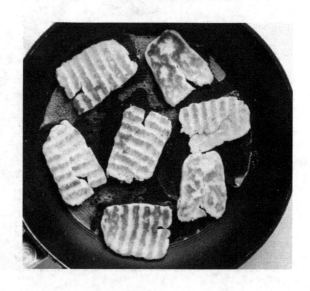

15. Toasted Bread for Bruschetta
(serves 8)

Ingredients:

1 garlic clove, peeled
Extra-virgin olive oil
1 (10 by 5-inch) loaf country bread with thick crust, ends discarded, sliced crosswise into ¾-inch-thick pieces
salt

Directions:

Adjust oven rack 4 inches from broiler element and heat broiler. Place bread on aluminum foil–lined baking sheet. Broil until bread is deep golden and toasted on both sides, 1 to 2 minutes per side. Lightly rub 1 side of each toast with garlic (you will not use all of garlic). Brush with oil and season with salt to taste.

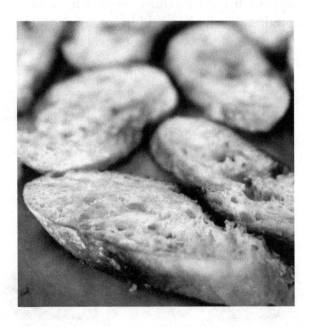

16. Bruschetta with Arugula Pesto and Goat Cheese
(serves 10)

Ingredients:

5 ounces (5 cups) baby arugula
¼ cup extra-virgin olive oil, plus extra for serving
¼ cup pine nuts, toasted
1 tablespoon minced shallot
1 teaspoon grated lemon zest plus 1 teaspoon juice
Salt and pepper
1 recipe Toasted Bread for Bruschetta
2 ounces goat cheese, crumbled

Directions:

Pulse arugula, oil, pine nuts, shallot, lemon zest and juice, ½ teaspoon salt, and ¼ teaspoon pepper in food processor until mostly smooth, about 8 pulses, scraping down sides of bowl as needed. Spread arugula mixture evenly on toasts, top with goat cheese, and drizzle with extra oil to taste. Serve.

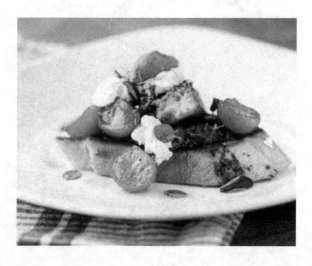

17. Bruschetta with Black Olive Pesto, Ricotta, and Basil
(serves 8)

Ingredients:

¾ cup pitted kalamata olives
1 small shallot, minced
2 tablespoons extra-virgin olive oil, plus extra for serving
1½ teaspoons lemon juice
1 garlic clove, minced
10 ounces whole-milk ricotta cheese
Salt and pepper
1 recipe Toasted Bread for Bruschetta
2 tablespoons shredded fresh basil

Directions:

Pulse olives, shallot, oil, lemon juice, and garlic in food processor until coarsely chopped, about 10 pulses, scraping down sides of bowl as needed. Season ricotta with salt and pepper to taste. Spread ricotta mixture evenly on toasts, top with olive mixture, and drizzle with extra oil to taste. Sprinkle with basil before serving"

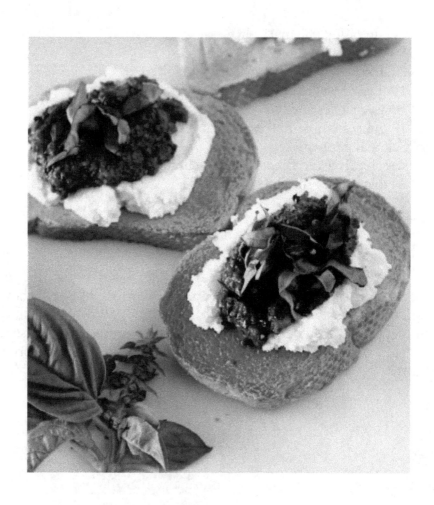

18. Bruschetta with Ricotta, Tomatoes, and Basil
(serves 10)

Ingredients:

1 pound cherry tomatoes, quartered
Salt and pepper
1 tablespoon extra-virgin olive oil, plus extra for serving
5 tablespoons shredded fresh basil
10 ounces whole-milk ricotta cheese
1 recipe Toasted Bread for Bruschetta

Directions:

Toss tomatoes with 1 teaspoon salt in colander and let drain for 15 minutes. Transfer drained tomatoes to bowl, toss with oil and ¼ cup basil, and season with salt and pepper to taste. In separate bowl, combine ricotta with remaining 1 tablespoon basil and season with salt and pepper to taste. Spread ricotta mixture evenly on toasts, top with tomato mixture, and drizzle lightly with extra oil to taste. Serve.

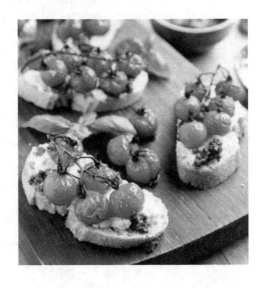

19. Bruschetta with Artichoke Hearts and Parmesan
(serves 8)

Ingredients:

1 cup jarred whole baby artichoke hearts packed in water, rinsed and patted dry
2 tablespoons extra-virgin olive oil, plus extra for serving
2 tablespoons chopped fresh basil
2 teaspoons lemon juice
1 garlic clove, minced
Salt and pepper
2 ounces Parmesan cheese, 1 ounce grated fine, 1 ounce shaved
1 recipe Toasted Bread for Bruschetta

Directions:

Pulse artichoke hearts, oil, basil, lemon juice, garlic, ¼ teaspoon salt, and ¼ teaspoon pepper in food processor until coarsely pureed, about 6 pulses, scraping down sides of bowl as needed. Add grated Parmesan and pulse to combine, about 2 pulses. Spread artichoke mixture evenly on toasts and top with shaved Parmesan. Season with pepper to taste, and drizzle with extra oil to taste. Serve.

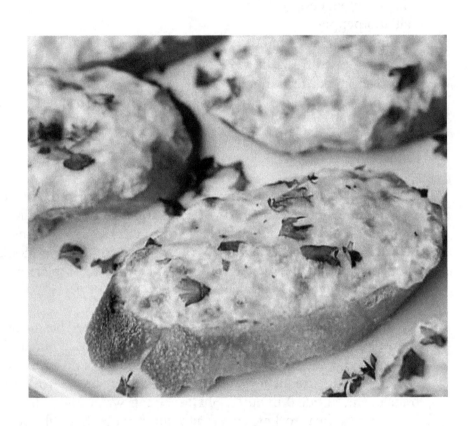

20. Stuffed Grape Leaves
(makes 24)

Ingredients:

1 (16-ounce) jar grape leaves
2 tablespoons extra-virgin olive oil, plus extra for serving
1 large onion, chopped fine
Salt and pepper
¾ cup short-grain white rice
⅓ cup chopped fresh dill
¼ cup chopped fresh mint
1½ tablespoons grated lemon zest plus 2 tablespoons juice

Directions:

1. Reserve 24 intact grape leaves, roughly 6 inches in diameter; set aside remaining leaves. Bring 6 cups water to boil in medium saucepan. Add reserved grape leaves and cook for 1 minute. Gently drain leaves and transfer to bowl of cold "water to cool, about 5 minutes. Drain again, then transfer leaves to plate and cover loosely with plastic wrap.

2. Heat oil in now-empty saucepan over medium heat until shimmering. Add onion and ½ teaspoon salt and cook until softened and lightly browned, 5 to 7 minutes. Add rice and cook, stirring frequently, until grain edges begin to turn translucent, about 2 minutes. Stir in ¾ cup water and bring to boil. Reduce heat to low, cover, and simmer gently until rice is tender but still firm in center and water has been absorbed, 10 to 12 minutes. Off heat, let rice cool slightly, about 10 minutes. Stir in dill, mint, and lemon zest. (Blanched grape leaves and filling can be refrigerated for up to 24 hours.)

3. Place 1 blanched leaf smooth side down on counter with stem facing you. Remove stem from base of leaf by cutting

along both sides of stem to form narrow triangle. Pat leaf dry with paper towels. Overlap cut ends of leaf to prevent any filling from spilling out. Place heaping tablespoon filling ¼ inch from bottom of leaf where ends overlap. Fold bottom over filling and fold in sides. Roll leaf tightly around[…]

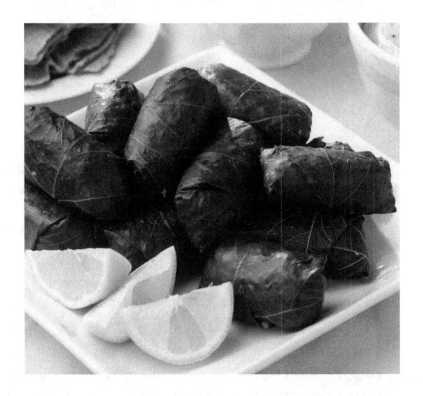

21. Sizzling Garlic Shrimp
(serves 8)

Ingredients:

1 bay leaf
1 (2-inch) piece mild dried chile, roughly broken, with seeds
1½ teaspoons sherry vinegar
1 tablespoon minced fresh parsley
1 pound medium-large shrimp (31 to 40 per pound), peeled, deveined, and tails removed
14 garlic cloves, peeled, 2 cloves minced, 12 cloves left whole
½ cup extra-virgin olive oil
¼ teaspoon salt

Directions:

1. Toss shrimp with minced garlic, 2 tablespoons oil, and salt in bowl and let marinate at room temperature for at least 30 minutes or up to 1 hour.
2. Meanwhile, using flat side of chef's knife, smash 4 garlic cloves. Heat smashed garlic and remaining 6 tablespoons oil in 12-inch skillet over medium-low heat, stirring occasionally, until garlic is light golden brown, 4 to 7 minutes; let oil cool to room temperature. Using slotted spoon, remove and discard smashed garlic.

3. Thinly slice remaining 8 garlic cloves. Return skillet with cooled oil to low heat and add sliced garlic, bay leaf, and chile. Cook, stirring occasionally, until garlic is tender but not browned, 4 to 7 minutes. (If garlic has not begun to sizzle after 3 minutes, increase heat to medium-low.)

4. Increase heat to medium-low and add shrimp with marinade. Cook, without stirring, until oil starts to bubble gently, about 2 minutes. Using tongs, flip shrimp and continue to cook until almost cooked through, about 2

minutes. Increase heat to high and add vinegar and parsley. Cook, stirring constantly, until shrimp are cooked through and oil is bubbling vigorously, 15 to 20 seconds. Remove and discard bay leaf. Serve immediately.

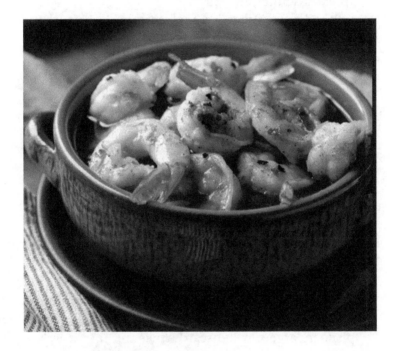

22. Mussels Escabeche
(serves 6)

Ingredients:

⅔ cup white wine
⅔ cup water
2 pounds mussels, scrubbed and debearded
⅓ cup extra-virgin olive oil
½ small red onion, sliced ¼ inch thick
4 garlic cloves, sliced thin
2 bay leaves
2 sprigs fresh thyme
2 tablespoons minced fresh parsley
¾ teaspoon smoked paprika
¼ cup sherry vinegar
Salt and pepper

Directions:

1. Bring wine and water to boil in Dutch oven over high heat. Add mussels, cover, and cook, stirring occasionally, until mussels open, 3 to 6 minutes. Strain mussels and discard cooking liquid and any mussels that have not opened. Let mussels cool slightly, then remove mussels from shells and place in large bowl; discard shells.

2. Heat oil in now-empty Dutch oven over medium heat until shimmering. Add onion, garlic, bay leaves, thyme, 1 tablespoon parsley, and paprika. Cook, stirring often, until garlic is fragrant and onion is slightly wilted, about 1 minute.

3. Off heat, stir in vinegar, ¼ teaspoon salt, and ⅛ teaspoon pepper. Pour mixture over mussels and let sit for 15 minutes. (Mussels can be refrigerated for up to 2 days; bring

to room temperature before serving.) Season with salt and pepper to taste and sprinkle with remaining 1 tablespoon parsley before serving."

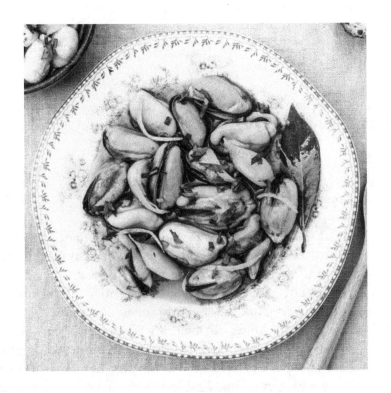

23. Stuffed Sardines
(serves 8)

Ingredients:

⅓ cup capers, rinsed and minced
¼ cup golden raisins, chopped fine
¼ cup pine nuts, toasted and chopped fine
3 tablespoons extra-virgin olive oil
2 tablespoons minced fresh parsley
2 teaspoons grated orange zest plus wedges for serving
2 garlic cloves, minced
Salt and pepper
⅓ cup panko bread crumbs
8 fresh sardines (2 to 3 ounces each), scaled, gutted, head and tail on

Directions:

1. Adjust oven rack to lower-middle position and heat oven to 450 degrees. Line rimmed baking sheet with aluminum foil. Combine capers, raisins, pine nuts, 1 tablespoon oil, parsley, orange zest, garlic, ¼ teaspoon salt, and ¼ teaspoon pepper in bowl. Add panko and gently stir to combine.
2. Using paring knife, slit belly of fish open from gill to tail, leaving spine intact. Gently rinse fish under cold running water and pat dry with paper towels. Rub skin of sardines evenly with remaining 2 tablespoons oil and season with salt and pepper.
3. Place sardines on prepared sheet, spaced 1 inch apart. Stuff cavities of each sardine with 2 tablespoons filling and press on filling to help it adhere; gently press fish closed.
4. Bake until fish flakes apart when gently prodded with paring knife and filling is golden brown, about 15 minutes. Serve with orange wedges."

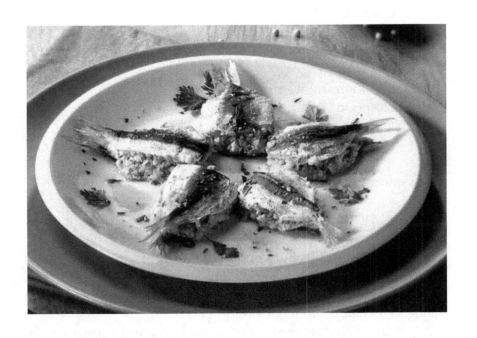

24. Chilled Cucumber and Yogurt Soup
(serves 6)

Ingredients:

5 pounds English cucumbers, peeled and seeded (1 cucumber cut into ½-inch pieces, remaining cucumbers cut into 2-inch pieces)
4 scallions, green parts only, chopped coarse
2 cups water
2 cups plain Greek yogurt
1 tablespoon lemon juice
Salt and pepper
¼ teaspoon sugar
1½ tablespoons minced fresh dill
1½ tablespoons minced fresh mint
Extra-virgin olive oil

Directions:

1. Toss 2-inch pieces of cucumber with scallions. Working in 2 batches, process cucumber-scallion mixture in blender with water until completely smooth, about 2 minutes; transfer to large bowl. Whisk in yogurt, lemon juice, 1½ teaspoons salt, sugar, and pinch pepper. Cover and refrigerate to blend flavors, at least 1 hour or up to 12 hours.
2. Stir in dill and mint and season with salt and pepper to taste. Serve, topping individual portions with remaining ½-inch pieces of cucumber and drizzling with oil.

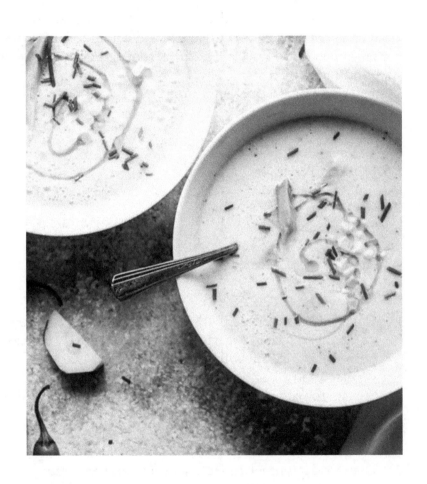

25. Classic Gazpacho
(serves 8)

Ingredients:

1½ pounds tomatoes, cored and cut into ¼-inch pieces
2 red bell peppers, stemmed, seeded, and cut into ¼-inch pieces
2 small cucumbers (1 peeled, both sliced lengthwise, seeded, and cut into ¼-inch pieces)
½ small sweet onion or 2 large shallots, chopped fine
⅓ cup sherry vinegar
2 garlic cloves, minced
Salt and pepper
5 cups tomato juice
8 ice cubes
1 teaspoon hot sauce (optional)
Extra-virgin olive oil

Directions:

1. Combine tomatoes, bell peppers, cucumbers, onion, vinegar, garlic, and 2 teaspoons salt in large bowl (at least 4-quart) and season with pepper to taste. Let stand until vegetables just begin to release their juices, about 5 minutes. Stir in tomato juice, ice cubes, and hot sauce, if using. Cover and refrigerate to blend flavors, at least 4 hours or up to 2 days.

2. Discard any unmelted ice cubes and season soup with salt and pepper to taste. Serve, drizzling individual portions with oil.

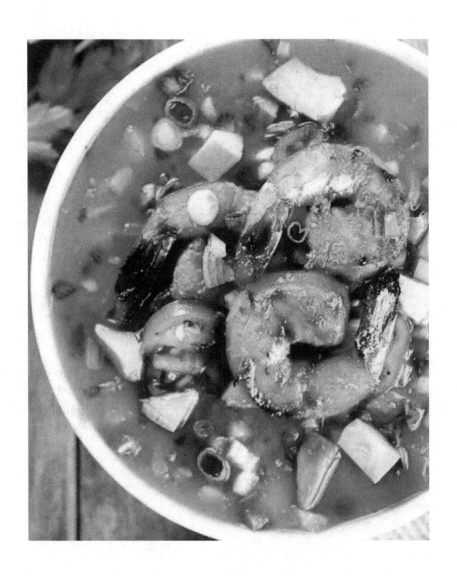

26. Classic Chicken Broth
(makes 8 cup)

Ingredients:

4 pounds chicken backs and wings
14 cups water
1 onion, chopped
2 bay leaves
2 teaspoons salt

Directions:

1. Heat chicken and water in large stockpot or Dutch oven over medium-high heat until boiling, skimming off any scum that comes to surface. Reduce heat to low and simmer gently for 3 hours.

2. Add onion, bay leaves, and salt and continue to simmer for another 2 hours.

3. Strain broth through fine-mesh strainer into large pot or container, pressing on solids to extract as much liquid as possible. Let broth settle for about 5 minutes, then skim off fat. (Cooled broth can be refrigerated for up to 4 days or frozen for up to 1 month.)

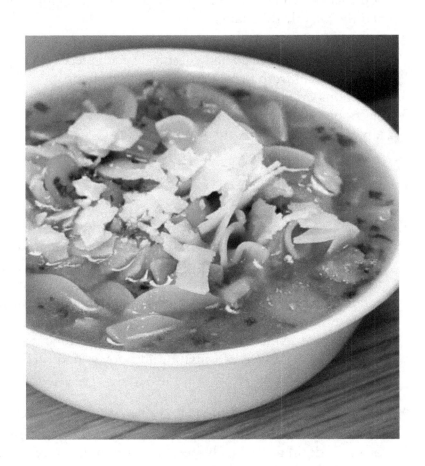

27. Vegetable Broth Base
(makes 1 cup)

Ingredients:

1 pound leeks, white and light green parts only, chopped and washed thoroughly (2½ cups)
2 carrots, peeled and cut into ½-inch pieces (⅔ cup)
½ small celery root, peeled and cut into ½-inch pieces (¾ cup)
½ cup (½ ounce) fresh parsley leaves and thin stems
3 tablespoons dried minced onion
3 tablespoons kosher salt
1½ tablespoons tomato paste

Directions:

1. Process leeks, carrots, celery root, parsley, dried minced onion, and salt in food processor, pausing to scrape down sides of bowl frequently, until paste is as fine as possible, 3 to 4 minutes. Add tomato paste and process for 2 minutes, scraping down sides of bowl every 30 seconds. Transfer mixture to airtight container and tap firmly on counter to remove air bubbles. Press small piece of parchment paper flush against surface of mixture and cover tightly. Freeze for up to 6 months.

2. TO MAKE 1 CUP BROTH Stir 1 tablespoon fresh or frozen broth base into 1 cup boiling water. If particle-free broth is desired, let broth steep for 5 minutes, then strain through fine-mesh strainer.

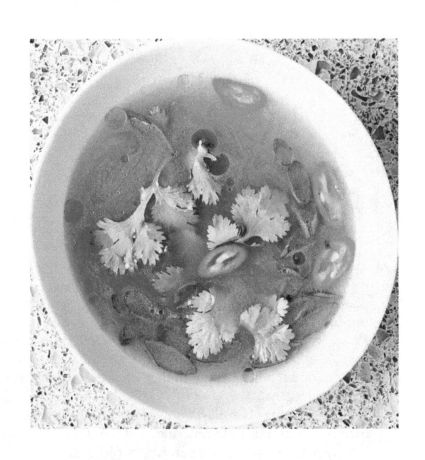

28. Roasted Eggplant and Tomato Soup
(serves 6)

Ingredients:

2 pounds eggplant, cut into ½-inch pieces
6 tablespoons extra-virgin olive oil, plus extra for serving
1 onion, chopped
Salt and pepper
2 garlic cloves, minced
1½ teaspoons ras el hanout
½ teaspoon ground cumin
4 cups chicken or vegetable broth, plus extra as needed
1 (14.5-ounce) can diced tomatoes, drained
¼ cup raisins
1 bay leaf
2 teaspoons lemon juice
2 tablespoons slivered almonds, toasted
2 tablespoons minced fresh cilantro

Directions:

1. Adjust oven rack 4 inches from broiler element and heat broiler. Toss eggplant with 5 tablespoons oil, then spread in aluminum foil–lined rimmed baking sheet. Broil eggplant for 10 minutes. Stir eggplant and continue to broil until mahogany brown, 5 to 7 minutes. Measure out and reserve 2 cups eggplant.
2. Heat remaining 1 tablespoon oil in large saucepan over medium heat until shimmering. Add onion, ¾ teaspoon salt, and ¼ teaspoon pepper and cook until softened and lightly browned, 5 to 7 minutes. Stir in garlic, ras el hanout, and cumin and cook until fragrant, about 30 seconds. Stir in broth, tomatoes, raisins, bay leaf, and remaining eggplant and bring to simmer. Reduce heat to low, cover, and simmer gently until eggplant is softened, about 20 minutes.

3. Discard bay leaf. Working in batches, process soup in

blender until smooth, about 2 minutes. Return soup to clean saucepan and stir in reserved eggplant. Heat soup gently over low heat until hot (do not boil) and adjust consistency with extra hot broth as needed. Stir in lemon juice and season with salt and pepper to taste. Serve, sprinkling individual portions with almonds and cilantro and drizzling with extra oil.

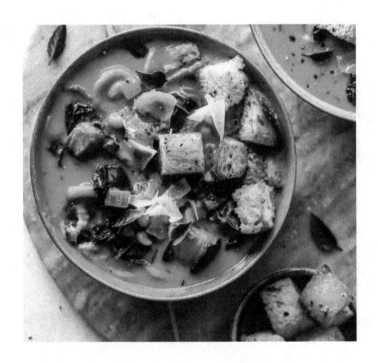

29. Provençal Vegetable Soup
(serves 6)

Ingredients:

PISTOU

½ cup fresh basil leaves
1 ounce Parmesan cheese, grated (½ cup)
⅓ cup extra-virgin olive oil
1 garlic clove, minced

SOUP
1 tablespoon extra-virgin olive oil
1 leek, white and light green parts only, halved lengthwise, sliced
½ inch thick, and washed thoroughly
1 celery rib, cut into ½-inch pieces
1 carrot, peeled and sliced ¼ inch thick
Salt and pepper
2 garlic cloves, minced
3 cups vegetable broth
3 cups water
½ cup orecchiette
1 large tomato, cored, seeded, and chopped
Passi di: America's Test Kitchen. "The Complete Mediterranean Cookbook". iBooks.
8 ounces haricots verts, trimmed and cut into ½-inch lengths
1 (15-ounce) can cannellini or navy beans, rinsed
1 small zucchini, halved lengthwise, seeded, and cut into ¼-inch pieces

Directions:

1. FOR THE PISTOU Process all ingredients in food processor until smooth, about 15 seconds, scraping down sides of bowl as needed. (Pistou can be refrigerated for up

to 4 hours.)

2. FOR THE SOUP Heat oil in Dutch oven over medium heat until shimmering. Add leek, celery, carrot, and ½ teaspoon salt and cook until vegetables are softened, 8 to 10 minutes. Stir in garlic and cook until fragrant, about 30 seconds. Stir in broth and water and bring to simmer.

3. Stir in pasta and simmer until slightly softened, about 5 minutes. Stir in haricots verts and simmer until bright green but still crunchy, about 3 minutes. Stir in cannellini beans, zucchini, and tomato and simmer until pasta and vegetables are tender, about 3 minutes. Season with salt and pepper to taste. Serve, topping individual portions with pistou.

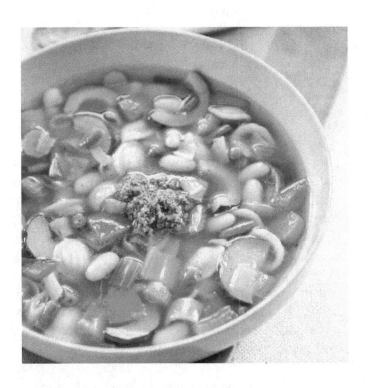

30. Turkish Tomato, Bulgur, and Red Pepper Soup
(serves 8)

Ingredients:

2 tablespoons extra-virgin olive oil
1 onion, chopped
2 red bell peppers, stemmed, seeded, and chopped
Salt and pepper
3 garlic cloves, minced
1 teaspoon dried mint, crumbled
½ teaspoon smoked paprika
⅛ teaspoon red pepper flakes
1 tablespoon tomato paste
½ cup dry white wine
1 (28-ounce) can diced fire-roasted tomatoes
4 cups chicken or vegetable broth
2 cups water
¾ cup medium-grind bulgur, rinsed
⅓ cup chopped fresh mint

Directions:

1. Heat oil in Dutch oven over medium heat until shimmering. Add onion, bell peppers, ¾ teaspoon salt, and ¼ teaspoon pepper and cook until softened and lightly browned, 6 to 8 minutes. Stir in garlic, dried mint, smoked paprika, and pepper flakes and cook until fragrant, about 30 seconds. Stir in tomato paste and cook for 1 minute.

2. Stir in wine, scraping up any browned bits, and simmer until reduced by half, about 1 minute. Add tomatoes and their juice and cook, stirring occasionally, until tomatoes soften and begin to break apart, about 10 minutes.

3. Stir in broth, water, and bulgur and bring to simmer.

Reduce heat to low, cover, and simmer gently until bulgur is tender, about 20 minutes. Season with salt and pepper to taste. Serve, sprinkling individual portions with fresh mint.

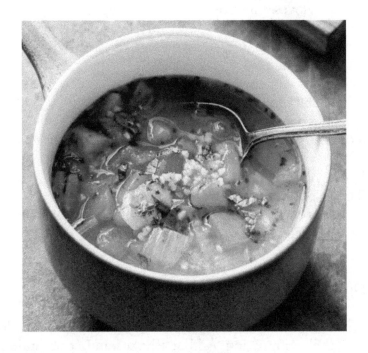

31. Artichoke Soup à la Barigoule
(serves 6)

Ingredients:

3 tablespoons extra-virgin olive oil
3 cups jarred whole baby artichokes packed in water, quartered, rinsed, and patted dry
12 ounces white mushrooms, trimmed and sliced thin
1 leek, white and light green parts only, halved lengthwise, sliced ¼ inch thick, and washed thoroughly
4 garlic cloves, minced
2 anchovy fillets, rinsed, patted dry, and minced
1 teaspoon minced fresh thyme or ¼ teaspoon dried
3 tablespoons all-purpose flour
¼ cup dry white wine
3 cups chicken broth
3 cups vegetable broth
6 ounces parsnips, peeled and cut into ½-inch pieces
2 bay leaves
¼ cup heavy cream
2 tablespoons minced fresh tarragon
1 teaspoon white wine vinegar, plus extra for seasoning
Salt and pepper

Directions:

1. Heat 1 tablespoon oil in Dutch oven over medium heat until shimmering. Add artichokes and cook until browned, 8 to 10 minutes. Transfer to cutting board, let cool slightly, then chop coarse.

2. Heat 1 tablespoon oil in now-empty pot over medium heat until shimmering. Add mushrooms, cover, and cook until they have released their liquid, about 5 minutes. Uncover and continue to cook until mushrooms are dry, about 5 minutes.

3. Stir in leek and remaining 1 tablespoon oil and cook until leek is softened and mushrooms are browned, 8 to 10 minutes. Stir in garlic, anchovies, and thyme and cook until fragrant, about 30 seconds. Stir in flour and cook for 1 minute. Stir in wine, scraping up any browned bits, and cook until nearly evaporated, about 1 minute.

4. Slowly whisk in chicken broth and vegetable broth, smoothing out any lumps. Stir in artichokes, parsnips, and bay leaves and bring to simmer. Reduce heat to low, cover, and simmer gently until parsnips are tender, 15 to 20 minutes. Off heat, discard bay leaves. Stir in cream, tarragon, and vinegar. Season with salt, pepper, and extra vinegar to taste. Serve.

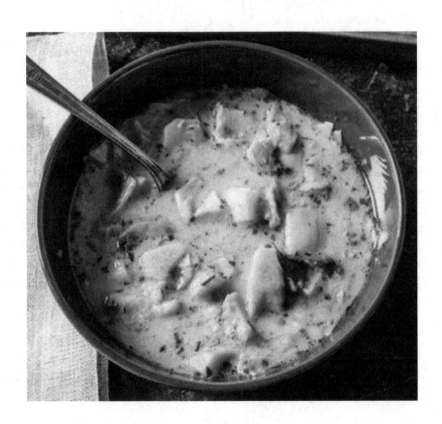

32. French Lentil Soup
(serves 4)

Ingredients:

3 slices bacon, cut into ¼-inch pieces
1 large onion, chopped fine
2 carrots, peeled and chopped
3 garlic cloves, minced
1 teaspoon minced fresh thyme or ¼ teaspoon dried
1 (14.5-ounce) can diced tomatoes, drained
1 bay leaf
1 cup lentilles du Puy, picked over and rinsed
Salt and pepper
½ cup dry white wine
4½ cups chicken broth, plus extra as needed
1½ cups water
1½ teaspoons balsamic vinegar
3 tablespoons minced fresh parsley

Directions:

1. Cook bacon in Dutch oven over medium-high heat, stirring often, until crisp, about 5 minutes. Stir in onion and carrots and cook until vegetables begin to soften, about 2 minutes. Stir in garlic and thyme and cook until fragrant, about 30 seconds. Stir in tomatoes and bay leaf and cook until fragrant, about 30 seconds. Stir in lentils and ¼ teaspoon salt. Cover, reduce heat to medium-low, and cook until vegetables are softened and lentils have darkened, 8 to 10 minutes.

2. Increase heat to high, stir in wine, and bring to simmer. Stir in broth and water and bring to boil. Partially cover pot, reduce heat to low, and simmer gently until lentils are tender but still hold their shape, 30 to 35 minutes.

3. Discard bay leaf. Process 3 cups soup in blender until smooth, about 30 seconds, then return to pot. Heat soup gently over low heat until hot (do not boil) and adjust consistency with extra hot broth as needed. Stir in vinegar and parsley and season with salt and pepper to taste. Serve.

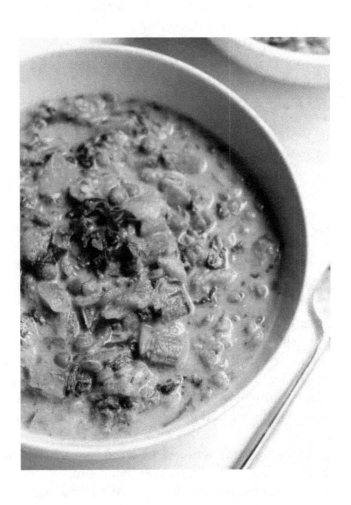

33. Red Lentil Soup with North African Spices
(serves 6)

Ingredients:

4 cups chicken or vegetable broth, plus extra as needed
2 cups water
10½ ounces (1½ cups) red lentils, picked over and rinsed
2 tablespoons lemon juice, plus extra for seasoning
1½ teaspoons dried mint, crumbled
1 teaspoon paprika
¼ cup chopped fresh cilantro
1 large onion, chopped fine
Salt and pepper
¾ teaspoon ground coriander
½ teaspoon ground cumin
¼ teaspoon ground ginger
⅛ teaspoon ground cinnamon
Pinch cayenne pepper
1 tablespoon tomato paste
1 garlic clove, minced

Directions:

1. Heat 2 tablespoons oil in large saucepan over medium heat until shimmering. Add onion and 1 teaspoon salt and cook, stirring occasionally, until softened, about 5 minutes. Stir in coriander, cumin, ginger, cinnamon, ¼ teaspoon pepper, and cayenne and cook until fragrant, about 2 minutes. Stir in tomato paste and garlic and cook for 1 minute.

2. 2. Stir in broth, water, and lentils and bring to vigorous simmer. Cook, stirring occasionally, until lentils are soft and about half are broken down, about 15 minutes.

3. Whisk soup vigorously until broken down to coarse puree, about 30 seconds. Adjust consistency with extra hot broth

as needed. Stir in lemon juice and season with salt and extra lemon juice to taste. Cover and keep warm.

4. Heat remaining 2 tablespoons oil in small skillet over medium heat until shimmering. Off heat, stir in mint and paprika. Serve soup, drizzling individual portions with 1 teaspoon spiced oil and sprinkling with cilantro.

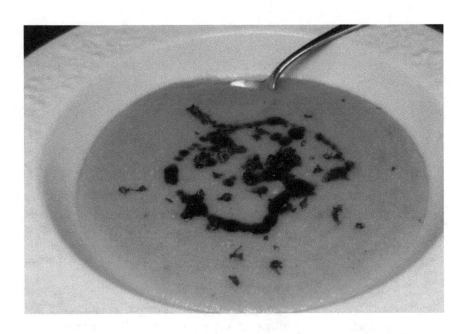

34. Moroccan-Style Chickpea Soup
(serves 6)

Ingredients:

2 (15-ounce) cans chickpeas, rinsed
1 pound red potatoes, unpeeled, cut into ½-inch pieces
1 (14.5-ounce) can diced tomatoes
1 zucchini, cut into ½-inch pieces
3½ cups chicken or vegetable broth
¼ cup minced fresh parsley or mint
Lemon wedges
3 tablespoons extra-virgin olive oil
1 onion, chopped fine
1 teaspoon sugar
Salt and pepper
4 garlic cloves, minced
½ teaspoon hot paprika
¼ teaspoon saffron threads, crumbled
¼ teaspoon ground ginger
¼ teaspoon ground cumin

Directions:

1. Heat oil in Dutch oven over medium-high heat until shimmering. Add onion, sugar, and ½ teaspoon salt and cook until onion is softened, about 5 minutes. Stir in garlic, paprika, saffron, ginger, and cumin and cook until fragrant, about 30 seconds.

2. Stir in chickpeas, potatoes, tomatoes and their juice, zucchini, and broth. Bring to simmer and cook, stirring occasionally, until potatoes are tender, 20 to 30 minutes.

3. Using wooden spoon, mash some of potatoes against side of pot to thicken soup. Off heat, stir in parsley and season with salt and pepper to taste. Serve with lemon wedges.

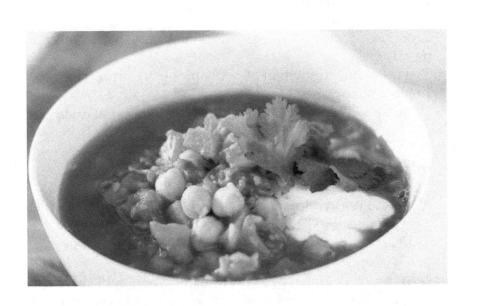

35. Greek White Bean Soup
(serves 6)

Ingredients:

6 cups chicken or vegetable broth, plus extra as needed
4 celery ribs, cut into ½-inch pieces
3 tablespoons lemon juice
1 teaspoon ground dried Aleppo pepper
2 tablespoons chopped fresh parsley
Salt and pepper
1 pound (2½ cups) dried cannellini beans, picked over and rinsed
2 tablespoons extra-virgin olive oil, plus extra for serving
1 onion, chopped
2½ teaspoons minced fresh oregano or ¾ teaspoon dried

Directions:

1. Dissolve 3 tablespoons salt in 4 quarts cold water in large container. Add beans and soak at room temperature for at least 8 hours or up to 24 hours. Drain and rinse well.

2. Heat oil in Dutch oven over medium heat until shimmering. Add onion, ½ teaspoon salt, and ½ teaspoon pepper and cook until softened and lightly browned, 5 to 7 minutes. Stir in oregano and cook until fragrant, about 30 seconds. Stir in broth, celery, and soaked beans and bring to boil. Reduce heat to low, cover, and simmer until beans are tender, 45 to 60 minutes.

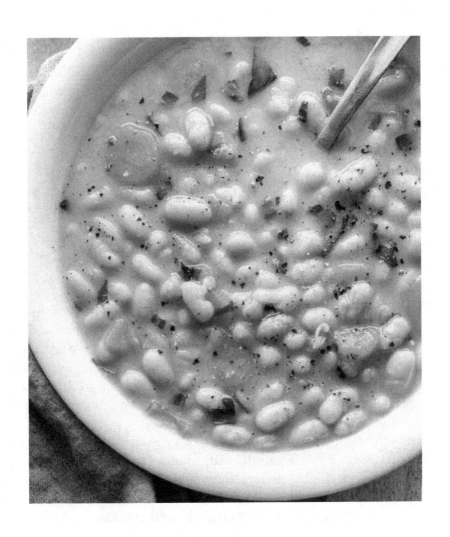

36. Spiced Fava Bean Soup
(serves 4)

Ingredients:

1 pound (3 cups) dried split fava beans, picked over and rinsed
6 cups chicken or vegetable broth, plus extra as needed
2 cups water
¼ cup lemon juice (2 lemons)
3 tablespoons extra-virgin olive oil, plus extra for serving
1 onion, chopped
Salt and pepper
5 garlic cloves, minced
2 teaspoons paprika, plus extra for serving
2 teaspoons cumin, plus extra for serving

Directions:

1. Heat oil in Dutch oven over medium heat until shimmering. Add onion, ¾ teaspoon salt, and ¼ teaspoon pepper and cook until softened and lightly browned, 5 to 7 minutes. Stir in garlic, paprika, and cumin and cook until fragrant, about 30 seconds.
2. Stir in beans, broth, and water and bring to boil. Cover, reduce heat to low, and simmer gently, stirring occasionally, until beans are soft and broken down, 1½ to 2 hours.
3. Off heat, whisk soup vigorously until broken down to coarse puree, about 30 seconds. Adjust consistency with extra hot broth as needed. Stir in lemon juice and season with salt and pepper to taste. Serve, drizzling individual portions with extra oil and sprinkling with extra paprika and cumin.

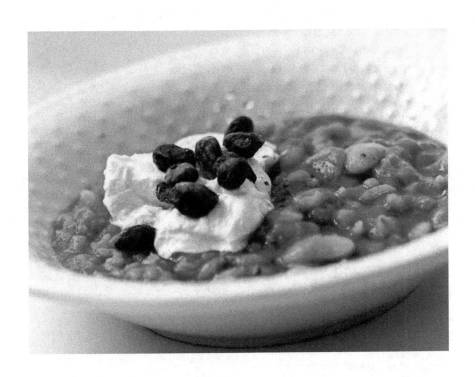

37. Spanish-Style Meatball Soup with Saffron
(serves 8)

Ingredients:

SOUP
1 tablespoon extra-virgin olive oil
1 onion, chopped fine
1 red bell pepper, stemmed, seeded, and cut into ¾-inch pieces
2 garlic cloves, minced
1 teaspoon paprika
¼ teaspoon saffron threads, crumbled
⅛ teaspoon red pepper flakes
1 cup dry white wine
8 cups chicken broth
1 recipe Picada
2 tablespoons minced fresh parsley
Salt and pepper"

Passi di: America's Test Kitchen. "The Complete Mediterranean Cookbook". iBooks.

MEATBALLS
3 tablespoons minced fresh parsley
1 shallot, minced
2 tablespoons extra-virgin olive oil
½ teaspoon salt
½ teaspoon pepper
8 ounces 80 percent lean ground beef
2 slices hearty white sandwich bread, torn into quarters
⅓ cup whole milk
8 ounces ground pork
1 ounce Manchego cheese, grated (½ cup)"

Directions:

1. FOR THE MEATBALLS Using fork, mash bread and milk together into paste in large bowl. Stir in ground pork, Manchego, parsley, shallot, oil, salt, and pepper until combined. Add ground beef and knead with your hands until combined. Pinch off and roll 2-teaspoon-size pieces of mixture into balls and arrange in rimmed baking sheet (you should have 30 to 35 meatballs). Cover with plastic wrap and refrigerate until firm, at least 30 minutes.

2. FOR THE SOUP Heat oil in large Dutch oven over medium-high heat until shimmering. Add onion and bell pepper and cook until softened and lightly browned, 8 to 10 minutes. Stir in garlic, paprika, saffron, and pepper flakes and cook until fragrant, about 30 seconds. Stir in wine, scraping up any browned bits, and cook until almost completely evaporated, about 1 minute.

3. Stir in broth and bring to simmer. Gently add meatballs and simmer until cooked through, 10 to 12 minutes. Off heat, stir in picada and parsley and season with salt and pepper to taste. Serve

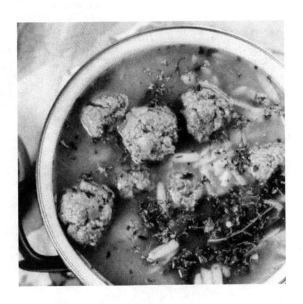

38. PICADA
(makes 1 cup)

Ingredients:

¼ cup slivered almonds
2 slices hearty white sandwich bread, torn into quarters
2 tablespoons extra-virgin olive oil
⅛ teaspoon salt
Pinch pepper

Directions:

Adjust oven rack to middle position and heat oven to 375 degrees. Pulse almonds in food processor to fine crumbs, about 20 pulses. Add bread, oil, salt, and pepper and pulse bread to coarse crumbs, about 10 pulses. Spread mixture evenly in rimmed baking sheet and bake, stirring often, until golden brown, about 10 minutes. Set aside to cool. (Picada can be stored in airtight container for up to 2 days.)

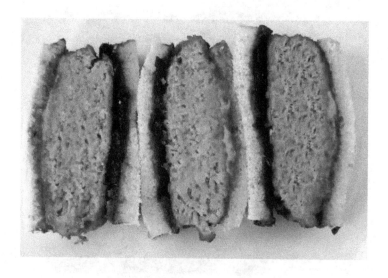

39. Provençal Fish Soup
(serves 6)

Ingredients:

4 garlic cloves, minced
1 teaspoon paprika
⅛ teaspoon red pepper flakes
Pinch saffron threads, crumbled
1 cup dry white wine or dry vermouth
1 tablespoon extra-virgin olive oil, plus extra for serving
4 cups water
2 (8-ounce) bottles clam juice
2 bay leaves
2 pounds skinless hake fillets, 1 to 1½ inches thick, sliced crosswise into 6 equal pieces
2 tablespoons minced fresh parsley
1 tablespoon grated orange zest
6 ounces pancetta, chopped fine
1 fennel bulb, 2 tablespoons fronds minced, stalks discarded, bulb halved, cored, and cut into ½-inch pieces
1 onion, chopped
2 celery ribs, halved lengthwise and cut into ½-inch pieces
Salt and pepper

Directions:

1. Heat oil in Dutch oven over medium heat until shimmering. Add pancetta and cook, stirring occasionally, until beginning to brown, 3 to 5 minutes. Stir in fennel pieces, onion, celery, and 1½ teaspoons salt and cook until vegetables are softened and lightly browned, 12 to 14 minutes. Stir in garlic, paprika, pepper flakes, and saffron and cook until fragrant, about 30 seconds.

2. Stir in wine, scraping up any browned bits. Stir in water, clam juice, and bay leaves. Bring to simmer and cook until

flavors meld, 15 to 20 minutes.

3. Off heat, discard bay leaves. Nestle hake into cooking liquid, cover, and let sit until fish flakes apart when gently prodded with paring knife and registers 140 degrees, 8 to 10 minutes. Gently stir in parsley, fennel fronds, and orange zest and break fish into large pieces. Season with salt and pepper to taste. Serve, drizzling individual portions with extra oil.

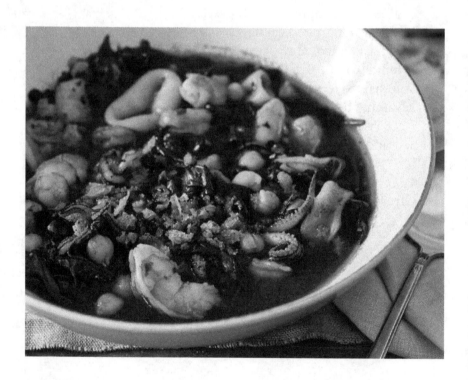

40. Basic Green Salad
(serves 4)

Ingredients:

8 ounces (8 cups) lettuce, torn into bite-size pieces if necessary
Extra-virgin olive oil
½ garlic clove, peeled
Vinegar
Salt and pepper

Directions:

"Rub inside of salad bowl with garlic. Add lettuce. Holding thumb over mouth of olive oil bottle to control flow, slowly drizzle lettuce with small amount of oil. Toss greens very gently. Continue to drizzle with oil and toss gently until greens are lightly coated and just glistening. Sprinkle with small amounts of vinegar, salt, and pepper to taste and toss gently to coat. Serve.

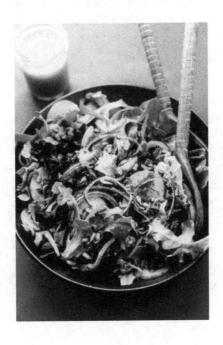

41. Green Salad with Marcona Almonds and Manchego Cheese
(serves 6)

Ingredients:

¼ cup extra-virgin olive oil
⅓ cup Marcona almonds, chopped coarse
2 ounces Manchego cheese, shaved
6 ounces (6 cups) mesclun greens
5 teaspoons sherry vinegar
1 shallot, minced
1 teaspoon Dijon mustard
Salt and pepper

Directions:

Place mesclun in large bowl. Whisk vinegar, shallot, mustard, ¼ teaspoon salt, and ¼ teaspoon pepper together in small bowl. Whisking constantly, slowly drizzle in oil. Drizzle vinaigrette over mesclun and gently toss to coat. Season with salt and pepper to taste. Serve, topping individual portions with almonds and Manchego.

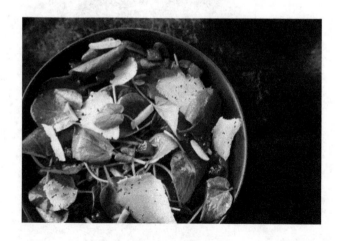

42. Tricolor Salad with Balsamic Vinaigrette
(serves 4)

Ingredients:

1 tablespoon balsamic vinegar
1 teaspoon red wine vinegar
Salt and pepper
3 tablespoons extra-virgin olive oil
1 small head radicchio (6 ounces), cored and cut into 1-inch pieces
1 head Belgian endive (4 ounces), cut into 2-inch pieces
3 ounces (3 cups) baby arugula

Directions:

Gently toss radicchio, endive, and arugula together in large bowl. Whisk balsamic vinegar, red wine vinegar, ⅛ teaspoon salt, and pinch pepper together in small bowl. Whisking constantly, slowly drizzle in oil. Drizzle vinaigrette over salad and gently toss to coat. Season with salt and pepper to taste. Serve.

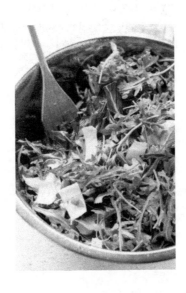

43. Green Salad with Artichokes and Olives
(serves 6)

Ingredients:

2 tablespoons white wine vinegar or white balsamic vinegar
1 small garlic clove, minced
Salt and pepper
3 tablespoons extra-virgin olive oil
1 ounce Asiago cheese, shaved
1 romaine lettuce heart (6 ounces), cut into 1-inch pieces
3 ounces (3 cups) baby arugula
1 cup jarred whole baby artichoke hearts packed in water, quartered, rinsed, and patted dry
⅓ cup fresh parsley leaves
⅓ cup pitted kalamata olives, halved

Directions:

Gently toss romaine, arugula, artichoke hearts, parsley, and olives together in large bowl. Whisk vinegar, garlic, ¼ teaspoon salt, and pinch pepper together in small bowl. Whisking constantly, slowly drizzle in oil. Drizzle vinaigrette over salad and gently toss to coat. Season with salt and pepper to taste. Serve, topping individual portions with Asiago.

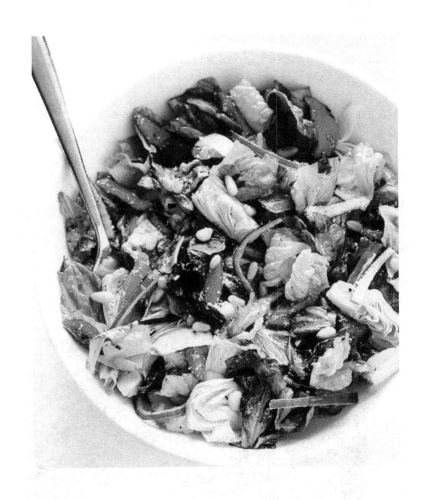

44. Classic Vinaigrette
(makes ¼ cup)

Ingredients:

½ teaspoon Dijon mustard
⅛ teaspoon salt
Pinch pepper
3 tablespoons extra-virgin olive oil
1 tablespoon wine vinegar
1½ teaspoons minced shallot
½ teaspoon mayonnaise

Directions:

Whisk vinegar, shallot, mayonnaise, mustard, salt, and pepper together in bowl until smooth. Whisking constantly, slowly drizzle in oil until emulsified. (Vinaigrette can be refrigerated for up to 2 weeks.)

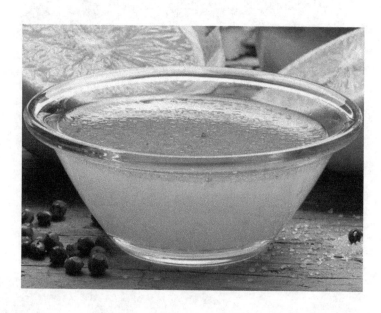

45. Walnut Vinaigrette
(makes ¼ cup)

Ingredients:

⅛ teaspoon salt
Pinch pepper
1½ tablespoons roasted walnut oil
1½ tablespoons extra-virgin olive oil
1 tablespoon wine vinegar
1½ teaspoons minced shallot
½ teaspoon mayonnaise
½ teaspoon Dijon mustard

Directions:

Whisk vinegar, shallot, mayonnaise, mustard, salt, and pepper together in bowl until smooth. Whisking constantly, slowly drizzle in oils until emulsified. (Vinaigrette can be refrigerated for up to 2 weeks.)

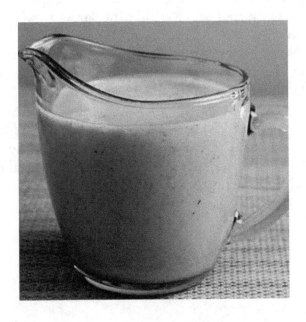

46. Arugula Salad with Pear, Almonds, Goat Cheese, and Apricots
(serves 6)

Ingredients:

½ cup dried apricots, chopped
3 tablespoons extra-virgin olive oil
¼ small red onion, sliced thin
8 ounces (8 cups) baby arugula
3 tablespoons white wine vinegar
1 tablespoon apricot jam
1 small shallot, minced
1 ripe but firm pear, halved, cored, and sliced ¼ inch thick
⅓ cup sliced almonds, toasted
3 ounces goat cheese, crumbled (¾ cup)
Salt and pepper

Directions:

1. Whisk vinegar, jam, shallot, ¼ teaspoon salt, and ⅛ teaspoon pepper together in large bowl. Add apricots, cover, and microwave until steaming, about 1 minute. Whisking constantly, slowly drizzle in oil. Stir in onion and let sit until figs are softened and vinaigrette has cooled to room temperature, about 15 minutes.

2. Just before serving, whisk vinaigrette to re-emulsify. Add arugula and pear and gently toss to coat. Season with salt and pepper to taste. Serve, topping individual portions with almonds and goat cheese.

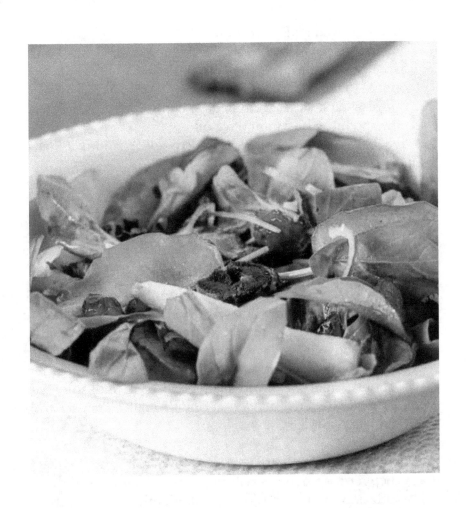

47. Asparagus, Red Pepper, and Spinach Salad with Goat Cheese
(serves 6)

Ingredients:

1 shallot, halved and sliced thin
1 tablespoon plus 1 teaspoon sherry vinegar
1 garlic clove, minced
6 ounces (6 cups) baby spinach
2 ounces goat cheese, crumbled (½ cup)
5 tablespoons extra-virgin olive oil
1 red bell pepper, stemmed, seeded, and cut into 2-inch-long matchsticks
1 pound asparagus, trimmed and cut on bias into 1-inch lengths
Salt and pepper

Directions:

1. Heat 1 tablespoon oil in 12-inch nonstick skillet over high heat until just smoking. Add bell pepper and cook until lightly browned, about 2 minutes. Add asparagus, ¼ teaspoon salt, and ⅛ teaspoon pepper and cook, stirring occasionally, until asparagus is browned and almost tender, about 2 minutes. Stir in shallot and cook until softened and asparagus is crisp-tender, about 1 minute. Transfer to bowl and let cool slightly.

2. Whisk vinegar, garlic, ¼ teaspoon salt, and ⅛ teaspoon pepper together in small bowl. Whisking constantly, slowly drizzle in remaining ¼ cup oil. Gently toss spinach with 2 tablespoons dressing until coated. Season with salt and pepper to taste. Divide spinach among plates. Toss asparagus mixture with remaining dressing and arrange over spinach. Sprinkle with goat cheese and serve.

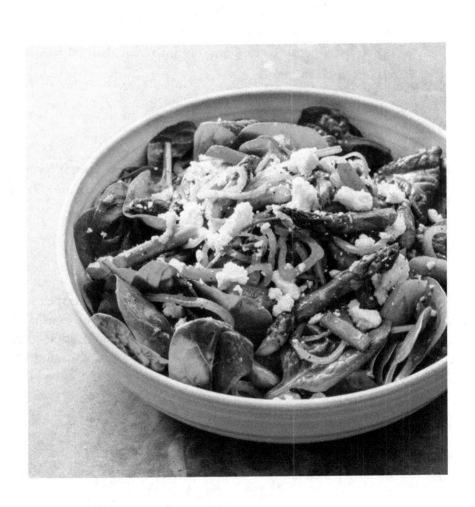

48. Bitter Greens Salad with Olives and Feta
(serves 6)

Ingredients:

½ cup pitted kalamata olives, halved
2 ounces feta cheese, crumbled (½ cup)
⅓ cup pepperoncini, seeded and cut into ¼-inch-thick strips
⅓ cup chopped fresh dill
2 tablespoons lemon juice
1 garlic clove, minced
Salt and pepper
3 tablespoons extra-virgin olive oil
1 head escarole (1 pound), trimmed and cut into 1-inch pieces
1 small head frisée (4 ounces), trimmed and torn into 1-inch pieces

Directions:

Gently toss escarole, frisée, olives, feta, and pepperoncini together in large bowl. Whisk dill, lemon juice, garlic, ¼ teaspoon salt, and ⅛ teaspoon pepper together in small bowl. Whisking constantly, slowly drizzle in oil. Drizzle dressing over salad and gently toss to coat. Serve.

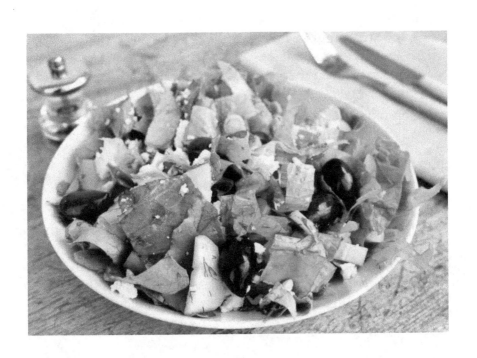

49. Mâche Salad with Cucumber and Mint
(serves 6)

Ingredients:

1 tablespoon minced fresh parsley
1 tablespoon capers, rinsed and minced
1 teaspoon minced fresh thyme
1 garlic clove, minced
Salt and pepper
¼ cup extra-virgin olive oil
12 ounces (12 cups) mâche
1 cucumber, sliced thin
½ cup chopped fresh mint
⅓ cup pine nuts, toasted
1 tablespoon lemon juice

Directions:

Gently toss mâche, cucumber, mint, and pine nuts together in large bowl. Whisk lemon juice, parsley, capers, thyme, garlic, ¼ teaspoon salt, and ¼ teaspoon pepper together in small bowl. Whisking constantly, slowly drizzle in oil. Drizzle dressing over salad and gently toss to coat. Season with salt and pepper to taste. Serve.

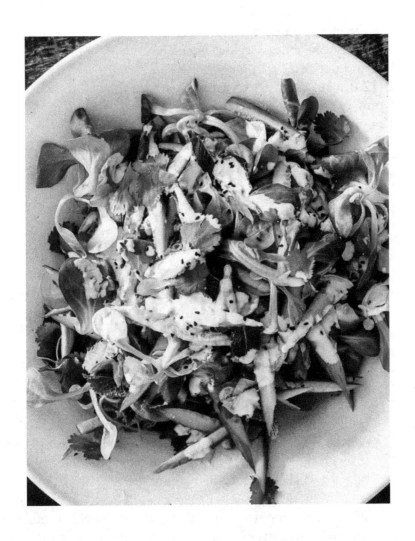

50. Seared Tuna Salad with Olive Dressing
(serves 6)

Ingredients:

1 garlic clove, minced
6 tablespoons extra-virgin olive oil
Salt and pepper
2 (12-ounce) tuna steaks, 1 to 1¼ inches thick
5 ounces (5 cups) baby arugula
12 ounces cherry tomatoes, halved
1 (15-ounce) can cannellini beans, rinsed
½ cup pimento-stuffed green olives, chopped
3 tablespoons lemon juice
1 tablespoon chopped fresh parsley

Directions:

1. Whisk olives, lemon juice, parsley, and garlic together in large bowl. Whisking constantly, slowly drizzle in 5 tablespoons oil. Season with salt and pepper to taste.

2. Pat tuna dry with paper towels and season with salt and pepper. Heat remaining 1 tablespoon oil in 12-inch nonstick skillet over medium-high heat until just smoking. Cook tuna until well browned and translucent red at center when checked with tip of paring knife and registers 110 degrees (for rare), about 2 minutes per side. Transfer to cutting board and slice into ½-inch-thick slices.

3. Whisk dressing to re-emulsify, then drizzle 1 tablespoon dressing over tuna. Add arugula, tomatoes, and beans to bowl with remaining dressing and gently toss to combine. Season with salt and pepper to taste. Divide salad among plates and top with tuna. Serve.

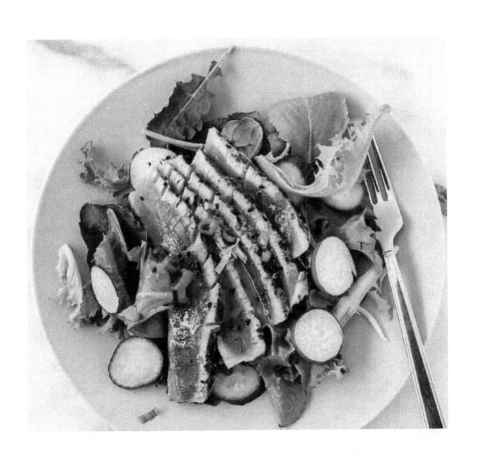

51. Loaf of Keto Pumpkin Bread

Ingredients:

1 1/2 cup Almond Flour
3 large Egg Whites
1/2 cup Pumpkin Puree
1/2 cup Coconut Milk (from the carton)
1/4 cup Psyllium Husk Powder
1/4 cup Swerve Sweetener
2 teaspoon Baking Powder
1 1/2 teaspoon Pumpkin Pie Spice
1/2 teaspoon Kosher Salt

Directions:

• Preheat oven to 350F
•I n a medium bowl sift all dry ingredients
• Put a container with 1 cup of water on the bottom rack of oven.
• Mix in pumpkin and coconut milk into dry ingredients and mix well.
• Whisk up egg whites until stiff. Slowly fold egg whites into dough.
• Place dough into a well greased loaf pan, then place into the oven and bake for 75 minutes.
•Let cool, then slice and serve!"

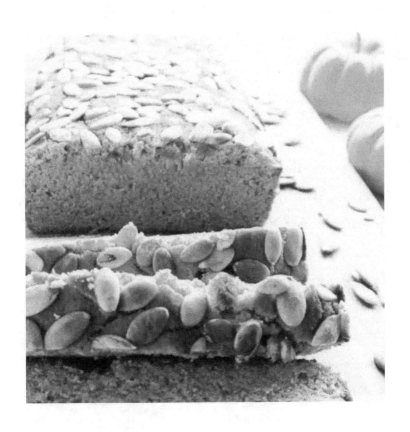

52. Scrumptous Keto Breakfast Muffins

Ingredients:

1 medium Egg
1/4 cup Heavy Cream
1 slice cooked Bacon (Cured, Pan-Fried, Cooked)
1 oz. Cheddar Cheese
Salt & Black Pepper

Directions:

• Preheat oven to 350 F

• In a bowl, whisk the eggs with the cream and salt and pepper.

• Spread into pam sprayed muffin tins, and fill the cups 1/2 full.

• Place 1 slice crumbled bacon to each muffin and then 1/2 oz cheese on top of each muffin.

•Bake for about 15-20 minutes or until slightly browned.

•Add another 1/2 oz of cheese onto each muffin and broil until cheese is slightly browned. Enjoy!

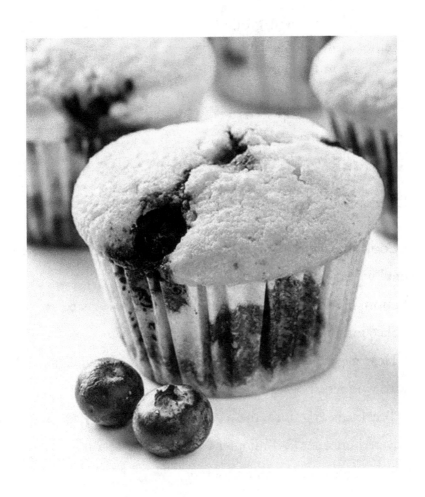

53. Keto Breakfast Mix

Ingredients:

2 tablespoon Sesame, ground
2 tablespoon Cocoa, dark, unsweetened
2 tablespoon Psyllium husk
5 tablespoon Coconut flakes, unsweetened
7 tablespoon Hemp seeds
5 tablespoon Flaxseed, ground

Directions:

• Cook spinach in a microwave safe bowl in microwave or steam until wilted

• Sprinkle with parmesan cheese and season to taste.

• Slice into bite size pieces and place on a plate.

• Heat a pan of simmering water, adding the vinegar and stir with wooden spoon to create a whirl pool.

• Break an egg into the center, turn of the heat and leave covered until set (3-4 minutes). Repeat with second egg.

• Place eggs on spinach and serve.

• Enjoy!

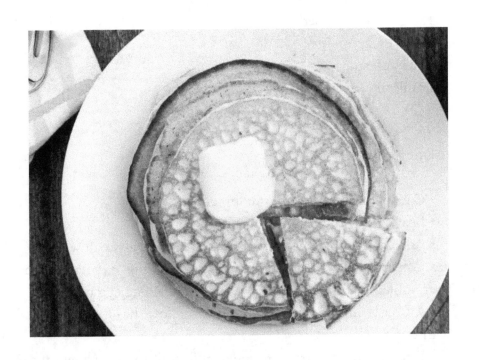

54. Quick & Easy Keto Spanish Omelette

Ingredients:

2 cups coarsely chopped vegetables
Pumpkin
Zucchini
Red capsicum
120 g fetta crumbled
3 eggs
¼ cup cream
2 tablespoons of olive oil

Directions:

• Cut and steam vegetables until tender, set aside.
• Beat eggs with cream, set aside.
• Add oil to a thick base fry pan and place on a very low heat.
• Mix in half of egg mixture to pan, put vegetables and crumbled fetta in pan and cover with remaining egg mixture.
• Cover with lid and cook on very low heat until cooked through.
• Place uncovered fry pan under grill until top of frittata turns golden brown."

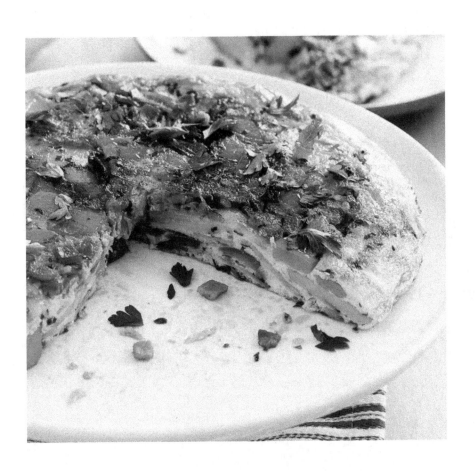

55. Keto Morning Breakfast Tea

Ingredients:

16 ounces water
2 tea bags
1 tablespoon ghee
1 tablespoon coconut oil
1/2 teaspoon vanilla extract
no carb artificial sweetener

Directions:

• Make the tea, set aside.

• In a different container melt the ghee

• Add coconut oil and vanilla to the melted ghee.

• Pour tea from mug into the magic bullet cup.

• Screw bottom on and blend until mixed thoroughly.

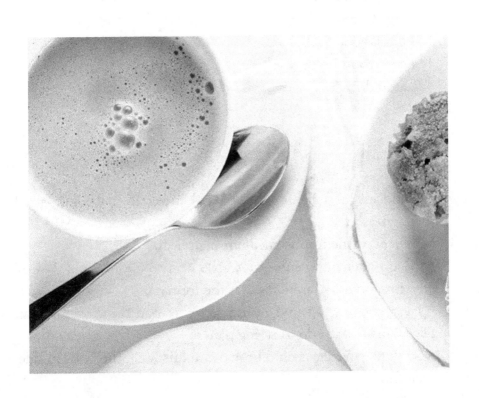

56. Keto Coconut Waffles

Ingredients:

1 cup Raisins
1 Tbsp ground Cinnamon
1 Tbsp Coconut Milk
1/4 cup Coconut Flour
1/4 tsp Baking Soda
1/4 tsp ground Nutmeg
4 Pastured Eggs

Directions:

• Blend all ingredients with a hand mixer in a medium-sized mixing bowl,.
• Preheat waffle iron to medium-high heat.
• Place batter into center of waffle iron to cover about 3/4 of area for about 3–5 minutes. For the topping:
• Heat coconut oil in a nonstick frying pan on medium heat. Slice banana and add to frying pan.
• Cook banana slices until brown and crispy on the bottom side, then flip.
• Add pecans to frying pan and lightly toast with the seared banana slices.
• Top over waffles or pancakes and serve.
• Enjoy

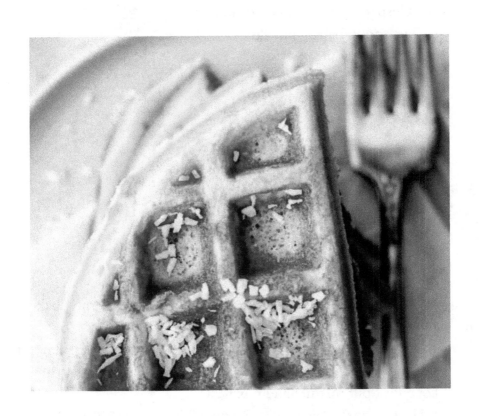

57. Keto Fluffy Coconut Flour Pancakes

Ingredients:

1/2 cup coconut flour
3 tablespoon granulated erythritol
1/2 teaspoon baking powder
1/2 teaspoon salt
6 large eggs, lightly beaten
1/4 cup butter, melted
1 cup almond milk
1/2 teaspoon vanilla extract
Additional butter or oil for the pan

Directions:

• Preheat oven to 200F.
• In a large bowl, beat together coconut flour, erythritol, baking powder, and salt.
• In a medium bowl, beat together eggs, melted butter, almond milk and vanilla extract. •Combine the egg mixture to the coconut flour mixture and mix well
• Heat a large skillet over medium high heat and brush with vegetable oil or melted butter.
• Pour two heaping tablespoons of batter onto skillet and spread into a 3 to 4 inch circle. Repeat until you can't fit any more pancakes into the skillet
• Cook until bottom is golden brown and top is set around the edges.

- Flip carefully and continue to cook until second side is golden brown.
- Remove from pan and serve warm
- Enjoy

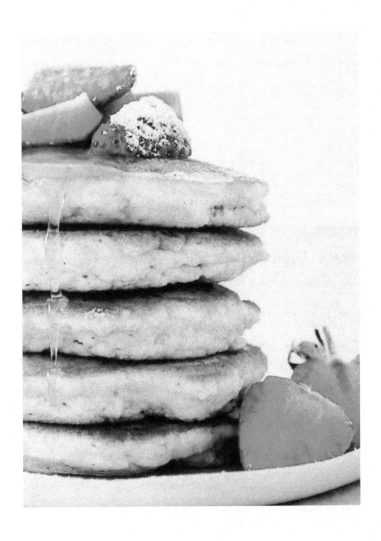

58. Keto Breakfast Banana Chia Seed Pudding

Ingredients:

1 Can Coconut Milk full fat

1 Medium or small size banana, ripe

1/2 teaspoon Cinnamon

1/2 teaspoon Salt

1 teaspoon Vanilla Extract

1/4 cup Chia Seeds

Directions:

• In a medium size bowl mash the banana until soft

• Combine the rest of the ingredients and mix until combined.

• Cover and place in the refrigerator overnight (or at least 2 hours)

• Enjoy!

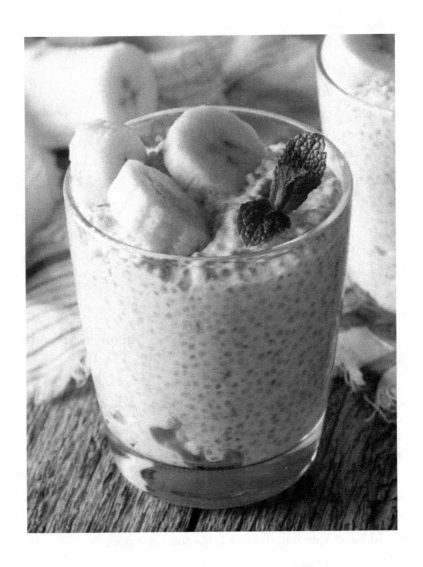

59. Keto Strawberry Rhubarb Parfait

Ingredients:

2 large eggs (free range or organic)
2 rings of large green pepper, approx. 1 inch thick
½ small red onion
1 cup fresh baby spinach
¼ cup sliced organic bacon
1 tbsp. ghee (or unsalted organic butter)
salt and pepper to taste

Directions:

• Cut peppers into two thick 1 inch slices.
• Grease a non-stick pan with half of the ghee or butter and add the pepper rings to the pan.
• Cook on one side for about 3 minutes.
• Crack an egg into each of the bell pepper rings.
• Sprinkle with salt and ground black pepper and cook until the egg white becomes firm. •When done, set aside.
• In a different pan, warm the remaining of the ghee or butter and add finely chopped red onion. Cook until slightly brown.
• Add sliced bacon and cook shortly.
• Add baby spinach and cook for another minute.
• Remove and enjoy!

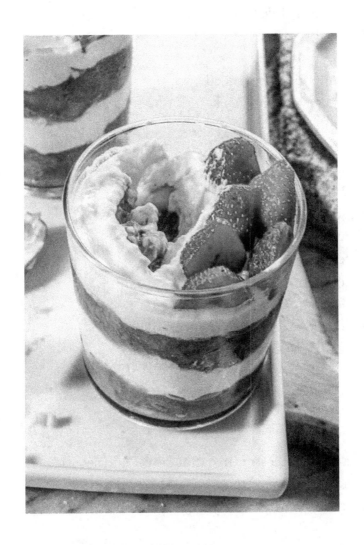

60. Keto Cinnamon "Oatmeal"

Ingredients:

1 cup Crushed Pecans
1/3 cup Flax Seed
1/3 cup Chia Seed
1/2 cup Cauliflower, riced
3 1/2 cups Coconut Milk
1/4 cup Heavy Cream
3 ounce Cream Cheese
3 tablespoon Butter
1 1/2 teaspoon Cinnamon
1 teaspoon. Maple Flavor
1/2 teaspoon Vanilla
1/4 teaspoon. Nutmeg
1/4 teaspoon. Allspice
3 tablespoon Erythritol, powdered
10-15 drops Liquid Stevia
1/8 teaspoon Xanthan Gum (optional)

Directions:

• In a food processor, rice cauliflower and set aside.
• In a pan over medium heat, add coconut milk
• In a different pan, crush pecans and cook over low heat to toast.
• Add cauliflower to coconut milk, bring to a boil, then reduce to simmer.
• Add in spices and mix together.

• Grind erythritol and add to the pan along with the stevia, flax, and chia seeds. Mix well
• Combine cream, butter, and cream cheese to the pan and mix again.
• Add xanthan gum (optionally) if you want it a bit thicker."

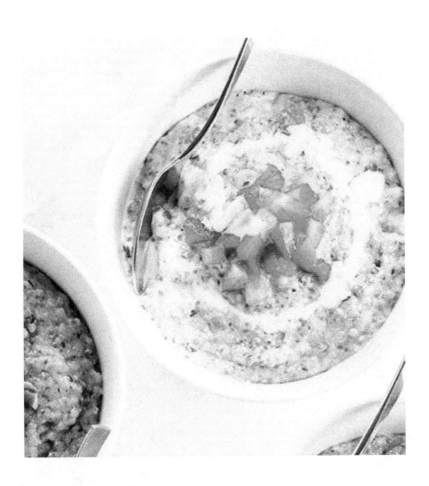